Evolve your emotions, Evolve through the Dimensions

CARLA SAVANNAH

Contents

CHAPTER 1

An Introduction

As I evolved within my Spiritual journey, I noticed people asking the same types of questions over and over again. How can I raise my vibration? What is my purpose? How can I manifest more and faster? These are all questions that I will address in this book.

By the time you've finished reading this book, you should have a clearer understanding of how to know and understand your purpose. You will have a clear understanding of what you need to do to raise your vibration, which will naturally result in manifesting more quickly.

Just a warning: I'm not a woo-woo fluffy type of teacher. I try my best to explain things in a way that is understandable for the average person. I explain things in layman's terms to make sure everyone gets it.

I want everyone to get more out of life. I want people to understand their potential, and I want people to realise their potential to light the flame within others.

So here is my first lecture. DO THE WORK! Don't skip ahead. Don't assume that just because you think you already know a lot about the world of energy and that you already are a high vibration being, you can just skip steps.

The ones who will gain the most from this and become the most successful Healers will be the ones who've put in the effort to do all the work that is this book.

If you start to feel lost at any point, then it's time to backtrack and go over the previous steps. You have to hold yourself accountable for your choice to do the steps and make the changes.

I'm literally spoon-feeding you all this information. I have researched the best of the best knowledge and combined it into this one basic, down to earth collective of information.

Happy Evolving!!

CHAPTER 2

In the beginning, there was darkness

In the beginning, there was darkness; then there was light. There was chaos; then there was order.

We have to remember that we came from nothingness. Then due to the right conditions, there was a big dispersing of energy. I will call this energy *light* for now. Projected light is merely white in appearance! When projected into water, glass, a form of matter or through you, it divides into a spectrum of light. You can see the light in contrast to the darkness, as shown in the image below.

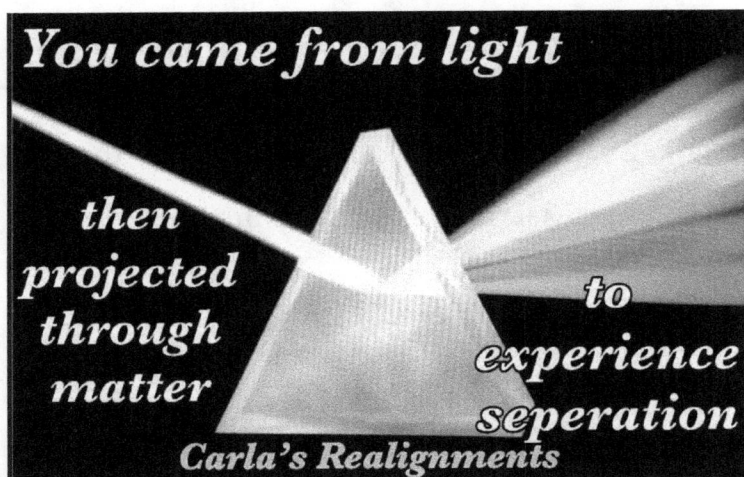

You are originally one light currently experiencing separateness projecting through the 3D dense matter world you live in. Within this separateness, you learn to see the colours of yourself that light the contrast of the darkness you were birthed from.

How else could you see and know your light without having the background contrast of darkness? It would be hard to see light within the light - like you can't show a fish what water is.

Light is a part of who you are. Darkness is the absence of light. Light is not the absence of darkness. You are Source energy learning about itself through individual units of itself. You are Source from Oneness experiencing itself in duality and separation.

Here's another way of looking at it. Consider the Big Bang Theory. One atom exposed to the right conditions exploded into many particles. Those particles then formed groups that began to vibrate together in patterns. These groups of patterns eventually formed stars, galaxies, planets, and eventually bacteria and cells that evolved into us today through trial and error. (If you're interested in reading scientific theories of the beginning of time, I suggest reading the trilogy *My Big Toe* by Thomas Campbell.)

There are mathematical codes and patterns all around you. Out of the chaos of this explosion came order and organisation of these cells. You could say the universe became conscious of its ability to create by forming and experimenting with grouping cells and matter together. This organisation is evident even within you.

You started life as an egg and a sperm, the egg being the ideal environment for the sperm's potential. They become one cell that began to divide and multiply until one group of cells formed a heart. The other group formed a liver, some formed lungs, and presto, here you are today. A human.

You are a universe of cells within a universe of cells becoming conscious of their ability to create and function as a whole organism. All the cells in your body function as a hive mind, like bees and ants do to create cities. From the micro-world of creators to the macro world of creators. You are God to one of the cells in your body.

So, what is the purpose of the universe? Number 1 is to expand and create that which begins as a chaos of cells. Number 2 to organise the chaos and form a functioning, orderly organism made of these cells. Number 3 is for this organism to become conscious of itself and its ability to create more cells and more patterns to create more organisms. The expansion continues, over and over it goes.

Eventually, the cells gain the ability to pollinate, explore and expand out to other planets, universes and galaxies. There's more power in numbers working together. If expanding and creating a self-conscious organism for further expansion is the ultimate purpose, how can we create this as a species?

We achieve this by uniting our species and working together. We are the individual cells, the neurological system or units of consciousness that makes up this vast organism we live in. How do we unite? Through loving and peaceful interactions. By creating a well functioning organisation amongst the chaos. By creating a conscious collective mind or harmonious hive mind, just like ants and bees that can create cities together.

Religions tried to connect people like this but keep failing in the long run. Do you know why religions and countries keep failing? Rather than encouraging individuals to become conscious of their independent power and ability to create and expand on their own, they created a hierarchy where humans had to rely on or be led by one entitled person. If that person doesn't care what happens to the majority, how will unity occur? We all know that it takes just one cancer cell to kill an entire organism. Perhaps that is why they don't want us to realise our power? In case we become that cancer cell. This is a fear-based, dysfunctional organism that breaks down individual cells' potential rather than helping individual cells evolve their potential. This is the complete opposite of expansion and creation. This would be imploding and deconstructing, in essence stepping backward towards chaos again.

Our future evolution depends on us becoming conscious individual cells that can also work as a collective group of cells. Knowing that we can expand individually, we can fulfil our unique potential, adding to the whole organism's functioning to grow together collectively.

How do we do this as individuals? Your purpose is to expand, create and evolve — the same as the universe's purpose, only on a smaller scale. Whatever allows you to do this to your greatest degree is what you should be doing. Experience and express yourself in as many ways as possible. Honour yourself as an individual. Create and build as much as you can while still having fun. A happy, self-fulfilled person doesn't feel the need to take anything from others. A happy human being is not a drain on others.

By integrating all of your inner light spectrum colours, you become one light again. Sages compare this to integrating all the Chakras (wheels of energy within the body).

The universal challenge for humanity is to find ways of connecting us all in a way that empowers us as individuals and us as the collective consciousness. The universe is already attempting to connect us through modern technology and the Internet. It's what we will *do* with that technological way of connecting that will be important. Will we use it for its designed purpose of connection and expansion? Or will we use it to create more separation and destroy our connection with each other?

Many people are disconnecting from social media and modern technology, which is creating two problems. It's creating division amongst people because some accept technology as beneficial while others reject it. Not dealing with our internal fears around social media is stopping people from learning "discernment". Discernment means filtering out what is true, useful information and what is false, useless information. By disconnecting from the world of information, you stop your intuitive abilities from developing around modern technology. In essence, some people ignore their worries about modern technology taking over their lives rather than finding solutions. A fractured society can't expand as one.

So you see, the purpose of life is *creation, expansion, becoming conscious of one's creations, evolving as one and expanding further as one.*

Many Spiritual teachers will tell you that love is the ultimate goal. I'm here to tell you the love is merely a stepping stone. Love is the in-between, necessary step that brings cells together towards a common goal— the desire to function together as a whole organism. We must have a feeling of love to desire a connection with others. A tailor must love each piece of his fabric to sew the pieces together to make a coat.

Unconditional love is the most significant milestone towards Oneness, but it isn't the final goal. Love is on the path towards even more expansion and towards more worlds. Yes, there are more worlds to come after this one.

I realise this is a lot to take in initially, but I promise it gets easier as the information starts to fall into place for you.

CHAPTER 3

The basics of 3D, 4D and 5D

Dimensions are complex, but here's a practical way of understanding them. Physical matter makes up 3D, emotions and thoughts make up 4D, and the thinking mind that creates thoughts, mathematical patterns, information and data makes up 5D.

When we die, we first shed our physical 3D body and move onto 4D. In 4D, Mediums often say we go through a life review where we revisit our life and identify what we want to learn and experience in our next lifetime. Here is where we shed our emotional body by experiencing all the joys and pains from different perspectives.

Once we shed our 4D emotional and thinking body, we are free to move onto the collective world of data, the 5D. 5D is also known as Spirit Realm, Higher Mind or Collective consciousness; just another step closer to the Source of all that is.

Inspiration comes in from the 5th dimension. 5D information has to be interpreted by the 4th dimension emotional world before we can then ground and experience it in 3D using the five basic human senses. Let me give you an example of how this works.

Imagine you receive a download of inspiration to bake a cake. Inspirational data comes from 5D. You then mentally analyse and emotionally feel whether you'd like to bake a cake. This reflection is 4D. You search your memory to see if you have the ingredients to bake a cake, whether you remember how to do it, whether you feel like doing it - this is all 4D thoughts and feelings. You then put these thoughts into action, start getting the ingredients together, and physically start making your cake. Making those physical actions is what's brings the inspiration to bake a cake into the Physical 3D world.

Here you have the perfect example of the process, from 5D inspiration being grounded by us creators in physical form. There's evidence of this all around you! Take the chair that you are currently sitting on. Someone received the idea or inspiration to make that chair. They then had to process and analyse how

17

they would do it intellectually before they created it physically. Can you see each dimension at work here? This cake analogy provides a perfect example of why humans are such powerful Creators. We can transfer inspiration, thoughts and feelings into physical experiences of dense matter through choice and action. We can translate information through the Dimensions.

This is an excellent reason not to be scared of the world of Spirit. If a human were to swat or wave at a spirit form, it would feel like a baseball bat has just hit them. As a human, you are much more physically dense and powerful than you think. The world of Spirit relies on us to feed them energy to survive (but let's save that for another book).

Why am I focusing on emotions within this book, you ask? Well, we are multidimensional beings experiencing ourselves in multiple dimensions at the same time. The 4th dimension is our bridge between our 5th-dimensional realm and our physical 3rd-dimensional realm. Our 4th-dimensional self, also known as the Ego (or subconscious, or matrix), is our *bridge* to our higher self, collective consciousness, Higher Mind, our Akashic Field, or our 5D self! I think you get the point. So many people have given all of these parts of self so many different names. I want you to know that, in essence, we are all talking about the same thing. What we call them doesn't matter. What is most important is that you understand the purpose of each of them and how they work.

Let's move on and take a closer look at our 4th-dimensional self, the Ego that everyone talks so badly about.

CHAPTER 4

The Ego

The Ego is the most primitive part of our brain, the reptilian part. Its job is to create predictable patterns, performing specific tasks like breathing, walking, keeping our heart beating on autopilot. It doesn't just deal with the physical aspect, though - it also tries to create predictable patterns around emotions.

An example of how the Ego creates emotional patterns can be seen in how some people may deal with traumatic events. Suppose you have experienced a traumatic event as a child, one around abandonment. The Ego will hold the signature of that trauma within your emotional energy body. As you grow up, every time you experience a sense of loss, this trauma is re-triggered as though you were still experiencing the trauma around abandonment. For example, a simple thing like your boyfriend going out with friends will bring back the trauma of your Father divorcing your Mother. You can see how someone can overreact in this situation towards their boyfriend. The Ego or emotional body won't let you forget the pain.

The Ego learns which experiences create pleasure and pain. It tries to keep you within predictable patterns to avoid pain. The Ego knows what worked in the past to induce pleasure, and it will encourage you to do those same things repeatedly. It makes sure you stay within your comfort zone and not venture into the unknown to avoid painful experiences. It appoints itself as the Governor of your physical experience. The Ego is designed to keep you physically safe.

When you try something completely new and out of your comfort zone, the Ego perceives that you've just done something crazy like jumping into a lake full of Crocodiles. In these types of situations, self-sabotage rears its ugly head in a desperate attempt to get you back into what's comfortable, predictable and safe.

Now let's not make an enemy of the Ego. We need to thank the Ego for playing this particular role of keeping us safe within our physical experience. It also has another vital function that we didn't forget when we incarnated into this physical experience - the desire to grow and expand. Essentially the energy of more, more more.

The Ego only knows how to do this at a physical level. So it thinks on the level of material matter! More money, more sex, more power, more chocolate. The Ego can only relate its need for more to its individual physical experience, not to a broader perspective of inclusion with others. It's essential to understand this because it's the key to the transcendence of the Ego.

Let's imagine a child who wants chocolate. If you were to give that child two chocolates, they would refuse to share. However, if you give a child an endless bucket of chocolates, they will be more than happy to give away some. Furthermore, if you allowed them to indulge in as much chocolate as their heart desires, I guarantee that child will eventually hit a point where it no longer desires chocolate the way it used to. The child will either feel sick or have satisfied its need for chocolate. After that, chocolate becomes a choice for the sake of a familiar experience. I tried this with one of my kids. Around Easter time, she had gotten so many chocolates I thought we would be eating chocolate for years. One day I just said, "Knock yourself out, eat as much as you want." And guess what? Today she is the only person I know that has self-control around chocolate, cakes and sweets. She's now 20 years old and still the same.

Another example is a woman who has wanted children her whole life, realising that dream and having as many children as she wants. Naturally, there will come a time when she has experienced the mothering role to its fullest and desires her freedom.

A mother who wasn't completely immersed in their mothering experience, who worked full time, or never had much time for her children is more likely to feel unfulfilled around her parenting experience. She may get clucky again to fully complete this emotional experience.

When you're able to experience a desire to it's absolute fullest potential within your physical experience, the Ego no longer attaches to needing this experience anymore. The Ego becomes detached or even bored because it knows it can fulfil its every physical desire or has had that experience and wants something new. Therefore, the secret to transcending the Ego is to give the Ego everything it desires at a physical level. Once the Ego knows that it can have and create everything it desires, it gets bored. Like a tame lion, it settles down and detaches from the adventure of seeking new experiences all the time.

A bored Ego with no physical needs or desires is of no threat to anyone else. Therefore, you are free to become an inclusive entity with your higher self by experiencing the world without attachment to anything. A freed Ego can then work as a team with your higher self. Seeing the Ego and the higher self working together to achieve goals is something special to experience. It's a state of non-resistance, just complete balance and harmony between your human self and soul self.

Our 4D self/Ego/emotional body (just like our Higher Self) must be allowed to explore what it can do, what it can feel, what experiences it desires within the parameters and rules of the 3D world. Remember *inspiration* is a suggestion from your higher self, like a whisper into the ear of your Ego (4D self), but the higher self NEEDS the Ego to become inspired for it to prompt the physical body to take physical action at a 3D material level. The Ego controls your endocrine system and hormones that trigger your physical body into taking action. Your Higher Self is in the constant process of finding the Ego's sweet spot to get it to co-operate.

To inspire the Ego to action and get it on board with your Higher Self's wishes, the Ego needs to feel motivated to take action. Since the 4D Ego's main desire is to feel good and stay safe, our Higher Self needs to communicate with the Ego in ways that achieve this. The Ego likes predictable patterns, and it worries about too many adventurous suggestions by the Higher Self. Quite frankly, the Higher Self thinks it can fly and is entirely free-spirited. The Higher Self doesn't understand the rules of the 3rd Dimension. It thinks, "Oh well, if you kill off this body, then we'll just have to get another one." In Spirit, there's no such thing as physical death.

The Dilemma comes when the Higher Self has whispered inspiration into the ear of the 4D Ego self. The Ego tries to control the inspired action by appointing itself the Governor of your Higher Self. It starts to create experiences of this inspiration using whatever tools it has to force things to happen. It uses manipulation, guilt, shame, fear, obligation, expectations, dominance, sacrifice, victimisation, dependence, inauthenticity, judgement, control, validation, and anger. Can you see where the majority of humanity is operating from? They are making decisions based on their 4th Dimensional self. The Ego has a strong sense of entitlement and is like a 2yo child stretching the rules. The Ego is learning how to find a WIN/WIN solution. This is entirely different from the common thinking of the Ego that usually says, "It's mine, it's all about me, and I want it now!"

The Ego filters all inspiration that comes in from our Higher Self, and thankfully it does that so well. Therefore, the Ego needs the motivation to venture outside of its comfort zone and ground things for us at a physical level. It needs to learn how to do this to combine both independent creativity and connective co-creating with others.

To summarise, the Higher Self, in essence, knows Connection and came from Oneness and is trying to experience its individuality in the 3D world. The Ego, however, understands only the separation of self and others. Therefore the Ego needs to learn what Oneness can feel like without losing its sense of individual uniqueness.

Unfortunately for the Higher Self, it's up to the Ego to decide how it implements the Higher Self's inspiration at a physical level. Both the Ego and Higher Self need to learn how to work together.

Suppose the Ego takes the inspiration from the Higher Self and warps it or does whatever it wants with that inspiration. In that case, a significant disconnect happens between the Higher Self and the 3D physical self that the 4D Ego self controls. The Higher Self starts to think, "Oh well, this being is not listening to me anyway, so what is the point in giving them any more inspiration?" It then disconnects further from its physical experience. People often ask me, "Why I can't access my intuition?" It is because of this disconnect. Most of the time, it's the Ego that's not wanting to listen to the Higher Self. The most common cause is that the person is so focused on connecting with their higher self rather than acknowledging their Ego/4D self.

CHAPTER 5

The emotions

In this chapter, I want to give you some information, a primer, if you will, to help you understand the rest of this book.

Your physical 3rd-dimensional self governs your first five basic human senses: touch, taste, smell, hearing and sight. Your hormones and endocrine system (the governor of your 3rd and 4th-dimensional selves) control your emotions. Your hormones put the energy in motion; they translate the energy generated from these hormones into physical action.

The 4th Dimension works like a vortex. It has a high vibrational peak and a low vibrational peak. The lower peak feels like quicksand pulling you down into 3D. The higher peak feels like a gentle propelling towards 5D.

The lower part of 4D is where the negative, dark entities reside and stuck Souls/Energies that haven't yet been able to transcend their darker shadow emotions. You will need to face your fears and demons to pass through this astral plane. Confronting the lower vibrational emotions happens here. Those who've transcended their disempowering emotions such as sadness, apathy, anxiety, shame, guilt, anger, depression and fear will be able to move beyond this point. Everyone needs to move through this point as it is the zone of transition which some religions used to call the Judgement Realm.

4D is where you experience deep wounded child emotions. Once you've overcome these powerless emotions, you move upward towards upper 4D and transition into 5D, the realm of empowering emotions like courage, flexibility, willpower, love, purpose, reasoning, acceptance and joy.

The vortex of 4D causes great movement towards either higher or lower. You never want to stay stuck here. Earthbound Soul's that have shed their physical body need to transition through here; it is where the life review begins to occur after someone dies. The Earthbound's job is to move through these emotions as fast as possible, so they don't stay stuck in this emotional loop in time.

Within this book, I'm going to detail the emotions you may be facing daily. I will teach you how to identify the emotion you are operating from and give you some activities to transition through that emotion towards higher vibrating emotions.

You see, most people are still operating from very low vibrational emotions. Lower emotions make your cells vibrate slower. Higher emotions make your cells vibrate faster or in a more patterned and rhythmic way. A person who may have had an occasional experience with high vibrating emotions may only operate from higher emotions twenty per cent of the time. The rest of the time, they are vibrating from lower emotions. This vibrational level translates into the quality of the choices they make. Twenty per cent may be high vibrational, but 80 per cent are low. What type of lifestyle do you think this person may have? Do you think they are in a state of happiness and abundance?

Why would it be important to identify where you are operating from? Well, it's simple. Are you manifesting what you want into your life? Are you living your life's purpose? Do you feel supported by your Universe? Do you have the ability to receive information from your Higher Self or guides easily? Do you get plenty of synchronicities or signs that you're on the right track in your life? If you answered no to most of these questions, then it's safe to assume you're not vibrating at as high a frequency as you may think.

When you are operating from a low vibe, ignorance is bliss. However, as you raise your consciousness levels and your vibe/frequency increases, the Universe starts to treat you differently. The Universe rewards you with positive karma. One of the laws of our

35

Universe is the law of attraction, which says like attracts like. Ge good deeds attract good deeds. The high vibe, highly conscious people, manifest faster and more significant results. Raising your consciousness/vibe doesn't just make you a powerful manifestor. Being conscious also makes the Universe interact with you differently. The Universe starts to hold you more accountable for your choices. The Universe treats you with the mentality of, "*You should have known better! Why did you go and do something that silly? Maybe you aren't as conscious as you thought you were.*" With consciousness comes power, and with power comes the responsibility of having that power.

The compulsory raising of consciousness is a way of avoiding power from falling into the wrong hands. People who gain a lot of the power begin to realise very quickly that they need to be even more responsible and more accountable for their actions.

For example, you wouldn't give a loaded gun to a two-year-old, would you? A two-year-old wouldn't have the consciousness that it takes to use a loaded gun wisely. Unfortunately, in some parts of the world, people still do give power to unconscious people. I'm hoping for this to change.

It is one of the motivations for writing this book - granted a somewhat selfish reason. I want to make sure that everyone who has access to power and manifesting abilities learns how to become more responsible. Part of me has to admit that not only am I doing this for humanity as a whole, but my motivating force is to create a safer world for our children. I hope that by raising humanity's consciousness, we will all take more personal responsibility for our choices, hence creating a safer world together.

Let's dive into the groups of emotions. Each group has a frequency or vibration higher than the other. We'll start with the group that has the lowest vibration.

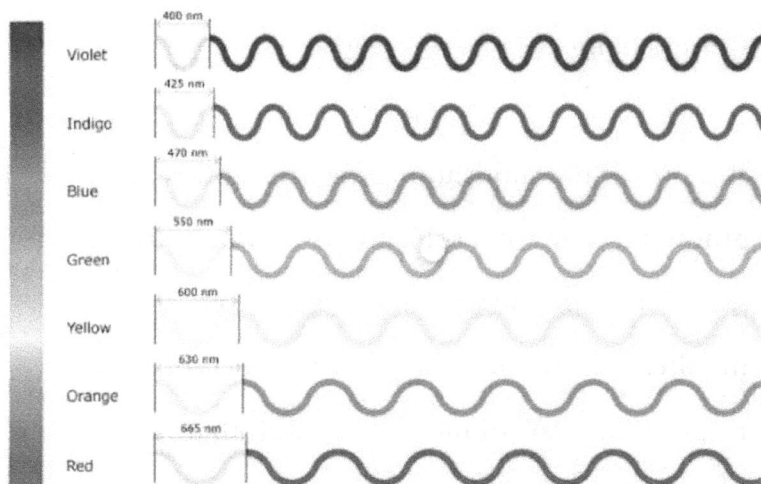

You can see how red has a lower frequency than the highest frequency, which is purple. These are often compared to the Chakras in the body. The lower root chakra starting at the bottom of our spine correlates with the colour red. It's our connection with the Earth and the low humming sound of the ground.

As we move up the spine, the frequencies get higher until we reach the Crown at the highest. I won't go into the Chakra system because the information is abundant for those who are interested.

My focus is on emotions and how these emotions' frequency associate with our body's vibrational levels. Whichever group of emotions we have mastered is the frequency we are operating from on the vibrational scale.

CHAPTER 6

The first group of emotions

The first group of emotions I want to talk about is
Disempowering Emotions such as regret, grief, guilt,
shame, fear, depression, hopelessness, loneliness, and
disconnection. This group is called disempowering
because these emotions keep people in a state of
powerlessness. A person operating from this state is a
victim of circumstances, environment, and people in
their lives. This person's survival is reliant on

absorbing energy from others or their environment. They often feel unsupported and, as a result, are unsupportive to life because most of the time, they have little energy left to give anyone else.

This person exists within the blame game. Everything is always everyone else's fault but their own. They are continually saying, "*My life is like this because he did this to me, or they did this to me, or it's because of my circumstances that I'm like this.*" They very rarely take personal responsibility for what is currently happening within their lives. They are always looking for someone to blame. This situation reminds me of an old Psychologist joke.

A client says to the Psychologist, "My life is a mess, and it's all my Mother's fault."

Psychologist: "Well, then, I'm sorry. I can't help you!"

Client: "What? Why not?"

Psychologist: "Go and tell your mother to come and see me so I can treat her for you to get better! It's useless to treat you if she's the one to blame for all of this. I'll fix her in the hope that it will fix you." Note how this person is taking no responsibility or accountability for their choices. It's essential to recognise where we are passing over blame.

Within this group, the person can fall into a sense of despair and have lost the will to live. They may spend much of their time sleeping or hidden away from society. They believe that they don't belong or fit in anywhere. This person may be in constant physical pain and suffering as the stagnation and lack of movement builds up stress spots and negative energy pockets within their body.

At their lowest point, this person doesn't even care for their basic needs such as cleanliness or proper feeding or looking after oneself. Sometimes they wish to check out, and sometimes the pain of being alive is more painful than considering death.

In some cases, a person in this group can fall into self-sacrificial martyrdom. They may believe that the only way to feel wanted or be loved is to do everything for everyone else. They are, in essence, handing over all their power to another person. They will go into a state of excessive service, desperately trying to gain some sort of significance from others. Their self-esteem is low. Within this low vibration, they genuinely believe that they are unworthy of more for themselves.

What this person needs

What this person needs is support. When they find this support, it will help them feel safe and secure. The above emotions make people believe that the world is unable to meet their needs. By seeking out the right resources, support and community, a person can feel like they are a part of something bigger again. The sense of belonging can return. When a person seeks safety, security and support, they re-establish their roots and move forward onto the next group of emotions more confidently.

Homework questions

Does this information resonate with you? If you feel these emotions most commonly, here are some questions to reflect on.

- Do I feel safe?
- How am I being supported?
- How can I feel more safe, secure or supported?
- Am I worthy of getting support?
- Do I feel wanted?

- How can I take better care of myself?

- What would make me feel more secure?

- Are my basic needs being met?

- Do I wash daily?

- How are my hygiene practices?

- What do I cling onto for security, and why?

- Who do I hand over my power to?

- Do I know the resources that are available to me?

- How can I find out what resources are available to me?

CHAPTER 7

The second group of emotions

The second group of emotions I want to talk about are the **Negative Controlling Emotions**. These include pride, anger, demanding, manipulation, hatred, jealousy, craving, disappointment, addiction, lust, controlling, sacrifice, greed, desperation, envious feelings and all subversions.

This group is referred to as the Negative Controlling Emotions Group because it is associated with actions or intentions that can be used to gain control or power over another person, situation, or environment.

Most of the time, these negative reactions stem from a fear that there is not enough in the world for this person. It's the desperation of wanting to grasp reality and is often born out of the lack mentality. Lack mentality means that there is a fear that there won't be enough for everyone and that this person will miss out if they don't forcefully take what they need or desire.

This person didn't like or realised that living in the previous disempowering emotions didn't serve many benefits. While they were operating from a place of disempowerment, they didn't have a sense of free will or control over their lives. Therefore, they had to find ways to start getting what they want. When operating within this group, a person desires to have their needs met; however, they haven't yet discovered healthy ways of achieving it. Instead, they use a motivating force such as anger, pride, aggression, or demanding to get what they want.

Anger can be a fantastic motivating force for people. When they stay in a passive and powerless state, most people find that they don't have the courage to stand up for themselves or demand what they want. However, once someone has stepped into a state of anger, suddenly, they dare to speak up and make sure their feelings are acknowledged. You can see how anger can be a tempting state to regularly fall into for someone who is continuously feeling disempowered, unacknowledged or unheard. Anger is just a shell to protect their more vulnerable, powerless emotions they don't want to show anyone. Anger, it turns out, provides a grand facade.

While a person residing within this group may start to take some actions towards fulfilling their needs, they still believe this can only be accomplished by other people or external circumstances. Thus, someone using this group of emotions is still a drain on society because they need to use some force or manipulation to meet their need demands. Jealousy provides an example of this. Imagine a girl has many personal insecurities around being loved because she felt neglected as a child. These insecurities may result in her possibly stopping her boyfriend from going out with his friends. She may become jealous when he speaks to other girls. She may manipulate him with threats of ending the relationship. These threats stem from her fear of being abandoned again. She expects her boyfriend to fulfil this need to be loved, and she uses emotional tactics to get what she wants—not realising that it's not his job to fix her. She's controlling him and taking away his free will to choose. Using an excess of control, this person believes in survival of the fittest and seeks to weed out the weak. They desire to create a hierarchy according to what they believe is right and wrong. It's all about them and what they can gain. They do what's best for their benefit in the long run, and they don't care whose toes they have to step on to get what they want.

This person comes across as selfish and without mercy or compassion—desiring to gain power over others. Love is conditional to them. An example of how they think is, "I will only love you if you do this for me. I will only love you my way under my rules." There is minimal compromise. If they look like they are trying to compromise, the underlying reason is always to get their way. These people only thrive in structured environments where they have complete control, or everything is entirely predictable.

What this person needs

This person needs to learn how to get what they want in ways that don't step or impinge on others' freedom. They need to learn healthy ways of getting their needs met. They need to be productive and creative in ways that don't drain and suck energy from others. They need to use their energy in constructive ways rather than in destructive ways. This person needs to start learning a certain amount of independence and self-control. A certain amount of selflessness can then begin to shine through. Above all else, they need to honour the free will of others.

Homework questions

Does this information resonate with you? If you feel these emotions most commonly, here are some questions to reflect on.

- What do I want or desire?

- What do I want to experience?

- What do I enjoy doing if I wasn't paid for it, getting any recognition for it or something in return for it?

- What inspires me?

- What am I afraid of changing?

- What am I afraid will happen if I try something new?

- What am I afraid will happen if I don't need anyone anymore?

- What am I afraid will happen if I lose control?

- I'll feel better when I do _____

- It makes me happy when I am _____

CHAPTER 8

The third group of emotions

The third group of emotions I want to talk about are
the **Power Emotions**. These include courage,
achievement, success, self-discipline, productivity, self-
confidence, empowerment, motivation, purpose,
commitment, reliability, strength, accountability, and
emotions around personal responsibility.

This group is called the Power Emotions Group because, for the first time, the person experiencing these emotions is not a drain on society. They understand that their ability to create and manifest comes from an internal power that no one else can give to them.

This person is taking full responsibility and accountability for all the choices that they are making. They understand that the universe is a feedback system-constantly giving direct feedback based on the choices we have made, not the choices others make. They are gaining a strong sense of self-awareness. They are happy to play their role in contributing to society rather than just looking out for their own needs. This person has something to offer society and starts to feel a sense of purpose as small as it may be. They have clear boundaries between themselves and others. They begin to do things for a greater cause.

These emotions are empowering emotions designed to create and accumulate energy from within. Once a person discovers that they no longer have to take energy from others, they can generate it from within themselves; they become self-sustaining. They access creative energy for themselves.

The beauty of this state of consciousness is that people start to realise that they have the Power to create changes in their lives for themselves. They no longer have to be limited by the patterns that raised them.

When in this state, someone who may have been abused as a child decides never to become the abuser. They desire to be better and are making choices around being better than what they were taught. They have stepped into their Power when they do this. They don't use the excuse "I'm this way because I was abused."

Often identified by their courage and willingness to try something new, these people are self-empowered and great motivators.

The downfall of this vibrational state comes if the person is without balance. This person can become negative in their excessive desire to create more and more energy now that they can access it for themselves.

When they are in an unhealthy state of these emotions, a person experiencing this consciousness level may become obsessed with work and have an overwhelming desire to succeed. They may obsess over goals, not caring who they step all over to get the job done. It is here there is a slight energy bleed from the previous grouping of emotions.

On the other hand, now being more responsible, they can sometimes take on excess responsibility for others. They always feel obligated to other people and are constantly apologising for not being good enough.

This consciousness level is a significant turning point for a person's evolution, simply because we never know what this person will do with their newfound power. Will they use it to benefit themselves only? Will they use it to benefit themselves and others? Or will they use this newfound way of creating energy to sacrifice themselves for others? I often see this happen within the Spiritual community. It is in this realm that people can become obsessive with being of service. Let me tell you that there is a big difference between being of service and becoming a servant. The Spiritual community can blur the two and make people feel bad if they aren't continually sacrificing themselves for others.

You may have realised that there is a bleed-over that seems to happen between each of the frequencies. This is not a black and white science. I'm merely giving you a foundation of energies to work with. This way, you can easily pick out where your family member, friend or client is operating from.

What this person needs

This person needs to learn how to create balance in their lives and establish clear boundaries around all aspects of their lives, be it family, relationships, work, finances or leisure. They now know that they are the powerful manifestors of their physical experience.

Therefore, they need to learn how to work with all their energy, utilising their ability to create healthy ways, not self-draining ways.

Homework questions

Does this information resonate with you? If you feel these emotions most commonly, here are some questions to reflect on.

- How can I establish boundaries?
- Do I believe that I have free will?
- How do I feel about responsibility?
- How might I be causing these current issues?
- Do I accept responsibility willingly?
- Am I holding myself accountable or responsible for my own life?

- What choices have I made that have led me to where I am now? Do I hold myself accountable for my choices?

- If I were to take responsibility for my life now, and what I've created, what might happen?

- Am I afraid of failure?

- Am I afraid of success?

- Which goals do I wish to achieve?

- What is my intention for my life?

- How can I become more self-disciplined?

- What action can I take today to move me towards my goal without taking other people's rights away?

- How can I gain more personal Power over myself?

- Do I allow my emotions to be heard?

- Do I understand that my emotions are my internal guidance system giving me signals all the time as to what's right and what's not right for me?

CHAPTER 9

The fourth group of emotions

The fourth group of emotions I want to talk about are

the **Connecting Emotions**. These include love, non-

judgement, forgiveness, acceptance, trust, co-

operation, neutrality, integration, compassion, and all

emotions designed to create connections.

This group is called the Connecting Emotions

Group because these emotions are based on creating

healthy, heartfelt connections with ourselves and others. Someone operating from this space is reasonable. They can see many perspectives and often look for a Win/Win solution to most situations. This person is co-operative and desires to find common ground with others. This person carries the energy of a typical counsellor or gentle advisor archetype. This person has a constant willingness to understand and connect with others. This person can get so caught up in their desire to connect that they may tend to lose a sense of self. The bleed over from the previous grouping is based on setting clear boundaries and not having their heart trodden on or taken advantage of.

Nothing is excluded when operating from this place; everything is being integrated. We become acutely aware of the world's polarity and duality and seek to find ways to connect it all. The Yin and Yang symbol describes this perfectly. We have both light and dark, but within the light, there is darkness, and within the darkness, there is light.

Let me share one of my favourite old shamanic stories of the White Wolf/Black Wolf. A Grandfather says to his Grandson, "*A fight is going on inside me. It is a terrible fight, and it is between two wolves. One is evil. He is full of anger, envy, sorrow, regret, greed, arrogance, self-pity, guilt, resentment, inferiority, lies, false pride, superiority, and ego. The other is good – he is full of joy, peace, love, hope, serenity, humility, kindness, benevolence, empathy, generosity, truth, compassion, and faith. The same fight is going on inside you – and inside every other person, too.*"

Grandson: "Which wolf wins?"

Grandfather: "*If you feed them right, they both win. If I only choose to feed the white wolf, the black one will be hiding around every corner, waiting for me to become distracted or weak and jump to get the attention he craves. He will always be angry and always fighting the white wolf. But if I* *acknowledge him, he is happy, the white wolf is happy, and we all win. The black wolf has many qualities: he is tenacious, courageous, fearless, strong-willed and has great strategic thinking that I need at times, and the white wolf lacks. But the white wolf has compassion, caring, strength and the ability to recognise what is in the best interest of all. You see, son, the white wolf needs the black wolf at his side. To feed only one would starve the other, and they will become uncontrollable. To feed and care for both means they will serve you well and do nothing that is not a part of something greater. Feed them both, and there will be no more internal struggle for your attention. And when there is no battle inside, then there is peace, and you can listen to the voices of deeper knowing that will guide you in choosing what is right in every circumstance."*

What this person needs

This person needs to learn, *how can I have me and have you too* thinking. They need to discover how to combine both to create balance within relationships. Understanding that your freedom ends where mine begins, and my freedom ends where yours begins.

Homework questions

Does this information resonate with you? If you feel these emotions most commonly, here are some questions to reflect on.

- If I was going to die tomorrow, what would have mattered to me the most?

- How can I feel more connected to those I love?

- What is most important to me?

- How can I show acceptance to all humans? How do I love more unconditionally?

- How do I show patience?

- How do I show compassion and nurturing?

- How can I offer healing to the world?

- How can I unite and bring those I love together? How can I open my heart to others?

- How do I feel about being vulnerable?

- How do I feel about surrendering to another person? What does intimacy mean to me?

CHAPTER 10

The fifth group of emotions

The fifth group of Emotions I want to talk about

are **Intellectual Emotions.** These

include understanding, intellectualising,

rationalising, objectivity, observing, reasoning,

studiousness, self-expression, witnessing, self-

awareness, vision, truthfulness. This group includes

feelings and emotions based on learning about the

seen and unseen world.

This group is called the **Intellectual Emotions Group** because, in this vibration, a person seeks knowledge and self-expression above all else. They can often appear to be very studious, as well as a teacher. This person desires to express themselves in the world, to be seen for what they have to offer as a unique individual. They are hungry for data and information.

Within this group of emotions, the desire to gather information can put someone on a path of endless studies, seminar attending and course-taking. This person can become insecure, thinking that they don't know enough to go about their life, job or business. They are driven by the need for clarity and confirmation that they are getting it right.

This person is developing their intellect in a way that doesn't allow them to be fooled easily. Often identified by their unique ability to see past a lie right to the truth or heart of a matter, this person has become a lie detector of sorts. They can pick up on people's true intentions and easily decipher when someone is lying to them.

In this level of consciousness, a person's intuition starts to develop as their observation skills become impeccable. The ability to slow down and analyse situations gives them enough of a gap between a stimulus and response to rationalise how they choose to react. It's often said that this is the difference between humans and animals. Animals are instinctual. They react quickly, without a thought. In contrast, humans have a small gap of time to think between what happens and how they react to what happens.

When this group of emotions is developing, a person can utilise and expand this small gap to rationalise the choice they are about to make.

This person utilises the emotions of 4D as an internal guidance system. They receive guidance more clearly and rationally and create a stronger connection between physical and energetic realms. The 3D physical self starts to trust that the 5D higher self will not put them in danger. The 5D higher self is beginning to trust that the physical 3D will not overreact on its animal instincts, creating a more trusting relationship between your multidimensional aspects of self. In essence, the division between our 3D self and our 5D self is not so big once we have fully activated our 4D self.

What this person needs

Discernment is the key factor here - the ability to perceive what is true for oneself instead of what's true for others or society as a whole—discerning what to say and what not to say. Discerning when it's time to speak and when it's time to listen, when it's time to learn and when it's time to teach. Discerning what is truth and what is fiction.

The risks of entering this grouping of emotions

The downfall that can come from having such vast knowledge now is Spiritual Ego can arise. This person needs to remain humble within this group of emotions so that they don't let their advanced education give them a sense of entitlement over others.

Another concern I have around this grouping of emotions is that there is a risk of someone switching

off, rejecting or denying their emotions altogether.
Many Spiritualists tend to desire to detach from the
physical self, whether they are aware that this is what
they are doing or not. In their extreme desire to raise
their consciousness and vibration, they remain in
their head all the time. They think that to be in
constant meditation is the only way to live a conscious
spiritual life.

Living only in the mind or astral realms is a blatant
denial of the physical body which you chose to come
and experience. By constantly disconnecting from
your body in this way, you are telling your body you
don't want to be in it. You are telling it you don't
want to have this physical experience by not being
present in your physical body.
Don't be surprised when your body starts to shut
down and you start having serious health issues.
You've disconnected from your biological system,

73

you're no longer animating it, so it starts to die off thinking that it's no longer needed. It's like a car that reached its maximum kilometres and is ready to be disposed of, replaced by a newer car. Devoid of emotions, you are ultimately an Artificial Intelligence. You're *intelligent* enough to intellectualise emotions, but you are not *biological* enough to FEEL them.

We aren't going up a step ladder as we go up the Dimensions. The goal is not to leave the 3D world and the 4D world behind as we move onto 5D upwards. The goal is to integrate all the Dimensions' knowledge and perspectives as we move upward and outward in perspective. Integration and knowledge of all is the goal.

Homework questions

Does this information resonate with you? If you feel these emotions most commonly, here are some questions to reflect on.

- How do I think others perceive me?
- How do others perceive me?
- How can I see this differently?
- Do I allow myself the time to self reflect?
- What do I want to learn more about? How can I educate myself on this?
- How can I understand more?
- How do I understand myself vs others?
- What do I desire to express or teach the world?
- Am I expressing myself authentically?
- How do I know what is me, and what's someone else?
- Do I feel heard?

- Do I feel understood?

- Do I know where I'm receiving my guidance from or who I'm connecting with?

- Do I have the ability to see various perspectives?

- Do I know the difference between sympathy and empathy?

- What does my current situation mean to me?

- What part of me is being ignored?

- How can I communicate better?

- How am I interpreting the world?

- What tool do I want to be on God's belt?

- How do I feel about my current qualifications?

- What do I have to offer the world?

CHAPTER 11

The spiritual Ego

One of the most significant challenges you will face as a Healer, Teacher or Seer is the Spiritual Ego. As our vibration raises and we become more powerful manifestors and healers, the sense of entitlement and lack of humility will show itself. Following are the signs signs of the Spiritual Ego showing up:

Magical Thinking: I'll just quit my job or jump off this cliff and trust that the Universe will catch me because I'm special and I shouldn't have to work.

Specialness: These are my gifts and abilities; let me show them off to you. I'm higher vibrationally and better than you. I've suffered more than you, so I have more experience.

Escapism: I'm too sensitive to be out in public. I don't like interacting with low vibration beings. I need to protect myself all the time.

Entitlement: I have more rights than you. I should be free to express myself. I need to be seen and heard by everyone to prove how much I know. I don't have to follow society's rules. I have the right to more freedom than you because I know better. This can also manifest as a lack of humility or forcing others to prove they are worthy of your time and the constant need to be right and win arguments.

Compassionless: You don't have the resources or knowledge, so I'm not going to waste my time with you. A you-brought-this-on-yourself mentality.

Hierarchy: Who have you trained with? Who is your teacher? Who do you know so that I can establish whether your information is validated by fame?

Fear of Ordinariness: I want to stand out rather than blend in. Ordinary is boring.

Impatience: Not trusting the process and wisdom behind the steady evolving. For example, I should have all the psychic abilities by *now*! I've worked hard enough and tried everything. I should have the abilities by now.

You can see how most of these can create a sense of separation between you and the world, which is the complete opposite of what Source wants.

The Human Ego is all about physical possessions and physical safety and survival. The Spiritual Ego comes from the upper 4D emotional/thinking energy body; it's slightly different because it's not worried about physical survival. It's more concerned about Dogmatic or Emotional/Mind Survival.

All lower-dimensional bodies have a duality/polarity/Ego to them. When you get into 5D upwards, there's less separation and more Oneness. While there's always a certain amount of separation until we reach the Oneness of 7D/8D upwards, the density is not as thick as you move up the dimensions. You could even say you have less individual free will as you move up the dimensions because you are subject to collective consciousness's direction and decisions in higher dimensions, not your individual unit of consciousness.

The opposite self or Ego is love and acceptance of all. No separation, just unity. Lack of Ego would be self not denied, like loving yourself and your reflection in the mirror at the same time. Both are you.

CHAPTER 12

The sixth group of emotions

The sixth group of emotions I want to talk about are
the **Joyful Emotions**. These include happiness,
laughter, joy, playfulness, optimism, fun, freedom,
and emotions that give a blissful state.

This group is called the **Joyful Emotions Group**
because it quite simply is all about feeling happy and
joyful. This group of emotions is also seen as the

Joker archetype. I feel as though this one needs very little explanation. When someone is operating from joyful emotions, it's very hard to get them down. Their light radiates outward, and they share their light no matter where they go. They can light up the room.

This person enjoys freedom and independence. They don't want to be tied down by anything that doesn't feel absolutely amazing and wonderful. They won't forgo the need to have fun while they do what they need to do.

What this person needs
Rarely does this person need anything. However, an essential lesson for a person who has reached this stage of their evolution is to remain compassionate for people operating from a lower energetic vibe.

This person needs to try their best to keep interacting with society. They tend to want to withdraw in the hope that they can maintain their high vibration away from others. Learning how to do this in the presence of others is their main challenge to overcome.

By holding a high vibrational frequency, they can raise the frequency of others within their vicinity without even needing to interact with them. Merely being within the presence of a person within this state of joy works like tuning forks. Their vibration will tune a like vibration in others.

The risks of entering this grouping of emotions
This person may be pulled down into guilt by society when they realise that not everyone knows how to create happiness for themselves the way they do. Someone in this constant happy state can be confronting to those who are more serious or

pessimistic. They may become withdrawn and disconnected from a society that doesn't wish to take personal responsibility for their happiness. And to be honest, by the time a person is firmly planted in this grouping of emotions, they have no desire to explain themselves to anyone. They just want to Be.

Homework questions

Does this information resonate with you? If you feel these emotions most commonly, here are some questions to reflect on.

- Am I having fun?
- How do I want to be remembered?
- What gives me joy?
- What or who makes me feel happy, and why?
- How can I add joy to the world?
- How can I share my happy vibes?

- How do I feel about those who present as being miserable and negative all the time?

- How can I feel freer?

- How can I free myself?

- What are my options?

- How can I create more options for myself?

- How can I create more time to do the things I love?

- What do I want to experience?

- What do I want to feel more of?

- What's on my bucket list?

- What have I had fun creating?

- What kind of results have I gotten from my actions?

- What kind of feedback is the universe giving me?

- Do I have a sense of obligation towards someone or thing?

CHAPTER 13

The seventh group of emotions

The seventh group of emotions I want to talk about

are the **Peaceful Emotions**. These include

peacefulness, calmness, stillness, unconditional love,

introspection, observation, quietness, contentment,

awareness, reflection, consciousness, enlightenment,

surrender, the silence of the mind and emotions that

accept all that is.

This person sees perfection and completeness in all that is. They don't desire to change anything; they just want to BE! They believe in live and let live. Only from this stillness can new ideas be birthed. It takes us right back to the memory that in the beginning, there was nothing. There was only calm and peacefulness, and from that stillness, something new was brewing into the Big Bang that created us today.

What this person needs

This person needs absolutely nothing! All is good in the world, and the world is just perfect the way it is.

Just because you are enlightened doesn't mean you stop living everyday life, washing the dishes or doing the laundry. Many make the mistake of thinking that just because they are enlightened, awake, and conscious, they have bypassed the need to be responsible for their physical experience. This thinking distinguishes those who are enlightened and those who aren't.

Enlightenment doesn't mean that you've transcended the needs of your human experience; it means you've integrated it. In Psychology, this is called self-actualisation or self-realisation. The enlightened person still washes clothes, washes dishes and walks the dog. The only difference is that the unenlightened person does it out of obligation and necessity. In contrast, an enlightened person does it with joy, fun and presence.

It's such a pleasure to watch an enlightened person do something as simple as washing the dishes because each time they do it, it's like the first time. They're like a child experiencing something new and exciting. That's how present they are. They are grateful just to have the physical experience of washing the dishes.

Homework questions

Does this information resonate with you? If you feel these emotions most commonly, here are some questions to reflect on.

- Do I feel at peace?
- Do I see the world as perfect?
- Am I grateful?
- Am I harmonious and peaceful?
- Do I know who I am?
- Do I understand that I am an eternal being, and physical death is not death at all?
- Have I come to terms with Physical Death?
- How do I feel about living?

- How can I contribute to the world if I were to stay?

- Do I see God in everything and everyone?

- Do I feel God in every moment?

- Do I have full access to the information of all that is?

- Do I have the ability to access my own Akashic Records.

CHAPTER 14

The differing levels of Consciousness

As you can see, many emotions drive people to make life choices based on the group of emotions they are operating from. If you are interested in another resource for learning more about emotions, I suggest *"Power Vs Force"* by Psychiatrist Dr David R Hawkins. He is the creator of the Map of Consciousness, based on Kinesiological testing. After many years in practice, Dr Hawkins determined that emotions have been scaled, and that is what the Map of Consciousness shows. It is well worth a read.

For now, let's look at everything you've learnt in this book using practical, everyday scenarios.

Example 1 - In the case of the loss of the family pet. Someone operating from the Disempowering Emotions group would go through a very lengthy grieving process that might be considerably longer than the average person. They may even try and find someone to blame for what happened.

Someone operating from the group of Controlling Emotions might become angry or mean towards the people around them. They may even find someone to take their emotions out on or blame.

Someone operating from the Power Emotions group might be very courageous and respond creatively by putting together a moment of farewell.

Someone operating from the group of Connecting Emotions may try to make sense of their loss. They may openly communicate their sorrow, desiring to understand what this loss will mean for their past and future without their pet. They will do their best to see everyone's perspective and address each person individually. They will logically rationalise their feelings rather than allowing them to consume them.

Someone operating from the Joyful Emotions group will look for all the positive ways their pet added to their lives. They will say things like, "Well, at least they aren't suffering any more". They will try to see the bright side of it all.

Someone operating from the Peaceful Emotions group may be the silent and present person there to offer unconditional love to whoever was most attached to the animal. They may react in this way because they most certainly aren't attached to anything of this physical realm. After all, they understand that there is no death.

Example 2 - Imagine being involved in a car accident, and the person you hit reacts with the following operating systems.

Someone operating from the group of Disempowering Emotions may have an anxiety or panic attack. They may come out of the car and start crying, unable to make any sense or calm themselves long enough to have a rational thought. This situation could go one of two ways; they may blame you for everything, or they will profusely apologise and admit fault for everything.

Someone operating from the Controlling Emotions group might become angry, start swearing at you and become physically confronting.

Someone operating from the Power Emotions group might admit responsibility if it was their fault and will approach you for negotiations.

Someone operating from the group of Connecting Emotions may immediately check if you are ok. They will be co-operative and tell you not to worry about it all as the insurance companies can take care of it. They may take extra care to check in on you later to make sure you are ok. There's no blaming here; they are simply resolution driven. They will stay rational. You may even become friends after this experience.

Someone operating from the group of Joyful Emotions will look for all the positives in the situation. They may say playfully, "Oh well, I needed a new car !" or, "Well, that was a silly thing to do". Either way, there is no animosity. All will leave happy and assured that the situation could be easily resolved.

Someone operating from the Peaceful Emotions group may calmly and politely exchange details without great opinion or emotion and move on quickly. But then again, I highly doubt a highly conscious person like this would ever be involved in a car accident. They just simply wouldn't attract this kind of drama into their lives.

Through this exercise, you can see how different people see their world and how they may be operating.

It is important to note that we use various operating systems based on different circumstances and situations. Let's take a closer look at what you are doing.

CHAPTER 15

Where are you operating from?

Let's take a look at each area of your life, starting with relationships. Think of a scenario that may have happened recently and ask yourself the following questions.

- What really upset me about what happened?

- What did it mean to me?

- How did I experience what happened?

- What do I think about what happened?

- What was the primary emotion that came up for me within this situation?

- What will I do differently next time?

Now answer these questions thinking about other areas of your life, such as career, finances, family, rest and relaxation, parenting, leisure and recreation, friendships, health, and sexuality. Take your time to *really* think through this activity. Don't rush it.

Which emotions came up the most? Which grouping of emotions did you find you were operating from the most? Where you able to find the deepest emotion? Where you able to pick some common patterns or regular go-to emotions for yourself?

If you found that you were operating from the Disempowering Emotions within most of the areas of your life, it means you need to focus on the questions for that section. They should lead you toward your next step, starting to focus on using your Controlling Emotions.

If you found that you mainly were operating from your Controlling Emotions, you need to revisit the questions in that section. It would help if you had some more practice in operating from the Power Emotions and so on. This practice allows you to move up the vibrational frequency scale slowly.

If you are operating from a state of Disempowering Emotions and Controlling Emotions, you are stuck firmly in the 4th Dimension. These emotions keep you in physical survival mode.

When you are operating from a state of Power Emotions, Connecting Emotions and Intellectual Emotions, you are operating within the 5th Dimension.

When you have integrated and accepted the lower emotions and are operating from a state of Joyful and Peaceful Emotions, congratulations! You are now operating on a 6th to 7th Dimensional level of vibration. Anything above the 7th Dimension means full integration with the Collective Consciousness. There is minimal separation between you and Source there. From 7D up, you become One with Source Consciousness again.

When you reach this state, you are becoming a powerful manifestor, but guess what? You don't even desire any of the power anymore. You will feel as though you are one with all, and you are no less than or more than. You are it. You are Creator.

CHAPTER 16

What is the Dark Night of the Soul?

While you are evolving through your emotions, you will find that you may come up against the Dark Night of the Soul. This is a very common phenomenon that happens to people doing lots of internal work on themselves.

It's a term often used within the Spiritual community to describe when someone is going through a transformation period. It's like a caterpillar going into the chrysalis, not knowing whether it will reemerge as a butterfly. The caterpillar is faced with the risk and fear of death to transform into a butterfly. This experience often happens when someone has had an initial trigger such as a mystical experience, traumatic event, near-death experience, deep healing work or a loss of someone they love. They go through a period where they question everything they have ever known to be real or meaningful. It's like a state of depression where a person may no longer feel as though there is any purpose or meaning in their lives.

It can feel like you're stuck drowning in quicksand, clueless as to how to get out. There's so much darkness, no clarity as to what the future will bring.

The most common emotions and feelings that come up are sadness, confusion, anxiety, numbness to life, and extreme lethargy. The things that once made you feel good no longer do. It's as if your natural spark has been blown out.

You may attract constant challenges, be it change of job, relationship break downs, health issues, financial issues and losses. You feel as though you just can't keep up with all the changes. You may sometimes suffer insomnia due to constant overthinking.

The Dark Night of the Soul can last anywhere from months to years, depending on how big you perceived the initial trigger to be. If psychological trauma or spiritual researching was the trigger, it should be dealt with and overcome slowly, like peeling away layers of an onion to minimise a prolonged state of depression. You must be delicate and compassionate with yourself.

During our current situation with this virus, I find many going through a "Death Bed" mentality. People are questioning what's important to them and whether they've lived their purpose! The best ways to overcome this state is to slow down, remain present and observe your feelings as they arise. Find the next best emotion that provides even just the smallest amount of relief and work your way up from there, with the intention of moving up on the emotional scale towards more positive emotions.

Understand that this is the path towards becoming a more awakened and enlightened version of yourself, becoming the butterfly. As you evolve, each time you go through it, it gets easier and quicker. You understand what's happening and simply treat it as just another episode of integration, transformation or upgrading from the old you into the new you. Think of it like an old iPhone learning to adjust to the latest software update. Trust that you won't malfunction; you just need time to adjust to the new knowledge and information coming in.

CHAPTER 17

Phases of change

What secret pleasure do you get out of staying the same? What personal pleasure do you get from not changing your circumstances? What satisfaction do you get with staying in your current situation?

Perhaps it's comfort. It may be security or significance. It may be a sense of appreciation or a desire to feel wanted, needed or loved. What drives you to do what you do? What motivates you to stay in your current patterns?

These questions can give you a heads up on why you struggle with change. I often ask my clients to defend all the reasons why they should keep doing what they have been doing. I ask them what secret pleasure they get out of staying the same? If they then remove that secret pleasure, guess what? Change becomes easy.

Most only change when put under extreme discomfort. Why not make changes within your life before things get so uncomfortable that you have no choice but to change? The universe always gives us a warning bell first. Unfortunately, most of humanity keeps pressing the snooze button repeatedly until a situation becomes life-threatening.

Here's what you need to know about change - it won't come easy!

So many people give up on change due to self-sabotage. The Ego makes them think that they will never reach their final goal. Think of it like you are contemplating going into a deep and dark tunnel. If you knew your greatest success was on the other side, that there was light at the end of the tunnel, would you persevere?

Let me explain the phases of change. Knowing these allows you to see that the self-sabotaging your Ego is doing is not to hurt you but because it is scared of change and unfamiliar territory. When self-sabotage is happening, you can stop it from taking control of you.

Here's what you can expect within each of these phases.

Phase 1 - The Mind Games Phase.

In this phase, you experience lots of internal resistance. You are considering change, but your mind is playing games with you. The Ego will use your mind against you. You will feel self-doubt, lack of clarity, discomfort and confusion around your desires. These feelings are your Ego attempting to stop you from leaving your comfort zone. It wants to stop you from venturing into any deep, dark, unpredictable tunnels. All these mind games cause procrastination and no real movement forward. No long-lasting changes can occur during this phase.

In this phase, you are forced to address issues such as laziness, blame, discomfort and anything that stops you from moving forward. The Ego does not want you to create any sort of momentum. Expect to come up against all kinds of resistance when you finally choose to enter the tunnel of change.

Phase 2 - The Freeze Phase.

Here is where you get stuck, thinking that you lack the resources to move forward. You will research, study and plan endlessly for a future event that is coming but never actually arrives. Not only do you doubt that you're ready, but your doubt itself attracts more doubt.

The subconscious mind/4th Dimension attracts drama with friends and family, arguments with your partner, unexpected bills and expenses, unforeseen health issues, and car and electrical equipment breakdowns. These are all issues that demand your attention immediately, and they are all there to distract you. They pull you off course and make sure your time runs out before you can create any kind of long-lasting changes.

Your Ego begins to worry that you are venturing out so far past your comfort zone that it can no longer keep you safe. The Ego says, "*What the hell are you doing! This is unfamiliar territory to me. How am I supposed to keep you safe here? Go back to your old patterns where it's safe and life is predictable!*" This situation is where the saying "Better the Devil you know, than the Devil you don't" originated.

This phase can be the longest to endure, but don't turn back now. Everything needs to change right here for you to become a vibrational match to your new life. In this phase, you will begin to shed away things and people that no longer serve a purpose in your new life. You are the caterpillar going into the chrysalis, unsure whether you will become the butterfly on the other side. You become one big vibrational mess. You are creating the new person you are becoming. You are no longer the person you once where, but you haven't yet become the person you aspire to be. This in-between freeze phase requires lots of patience, persistence and self-discipline.

Within this phase, you must address your issues around grief, loss, attachment, letting go, regret and forgiveness—the fear of losing everything to which you've become so attached. You risk getting stuck here because of your fear of letting go. You risk returning to what is safe. Things will become very interesting if you persevere through this very anxious phase and shed what is no longer needed.

Phase 3 - The Fight Phase.

When you reach this phase, you are on the verge of a huge breakthrough. Change is in the air. You've entered the deepest part of the tunnel, where you will experience extreme fear of uncertainty.

It's in fear of the unknown that you are faced with darkness, terror, sometimes even fear of death. You will feel extreme amounts of anxiety and adrenaline coursing through you. You are ready to fight at a moments notice but keep moving. Push through and overcome your deepest fears.

Prepare for Battle! Utilise the gift of pride, use the power of your anger, awaken the strength and courage within to confront what is there in the shadows and emerge on the other side victorious.

Phase 4 - The Confidence Phase.

You have defeated your demons in the shadows and think you are out of the woods. This is all an illusion. This phase is a mixture of exhaustion and a newfound courageous you. The spiritual Ego may arise within.

The universe may open up cues, clues, possibilities, synchronicities and opportunities for you.

You can finally see the light at the end of the tunnel and have a glimpse of what's awaiting you once you come out the other end. You think your work is complete, so you suffer the illusion that the universe will catch you every time you fall. You think you've done all the hard work now, and everything will magically unfold before you.

You desire to let go of the reins and handover responsibility to the universe. You may feel a sense of entitlement for all your hard work, but your job isn't over. You must persist towards the final phase.

Phase 5 - The Adaptation Phase.

Time to stabilise and get comfortable with the new you. You have gained new tools like clarity, self-discipline, responsibility, detachment, courage, determination and intuition. It's time to adapt, enjoy and utilise your newfound tools within.

It's time to create a new life full of courage, strength, stability, self-esteem, understanding, growth, acceptance, free will, peace, wisdom, balance, safety, trust, patience and FREEDOM.

This cycle begins anew each time you want to change. By this point, you've mastered it, and you move through the phases quicker and easier each time.

CHAPTER 18

Am I on the right path?

A common question I get asked is, "How do I know I'm on the right path?" It is a great question. My answer is that you experience very real signs and tangible results when acting in alignment with your higher self.

You see, Earth provides you with a great feedback system. The Universe is constantly in motion and provides you with an energy exchange to the energy you put out. This energy is never stagnant; it's always in flow. Whether you get favourable flow or negative flow in your direction is very dependent on the flow that you are giving out based on the choices you are making. The key energy to look out for is resistance.

There are two types of resistance. There is real resistance and false resistance. But first, let's look at what resistance is.

Resistance is when something isn't going your way or when things haven't turned out the way you expected them to. Some people interpret resistance as not being the right time. They say things like, "Maybe it wasn't meant to be?" or "Perhaps there is something wrong", or "It was the wrong path for me". Resistance can turn into stubbornness, and this is what the Ego wants.

You see, the Ego, your inner child/subconscious mind/robotic mind/primitive survival self/whatever you'd like to call it, likes old repetitive, predictable patterns. As soon as you start doing something new, the Ego wants you to stop. It thinks the unknown is scary, and it doesn't like you trying to change everything. So, it's not surprising that it creates some sort of self-sabotage to stop this new action when you tried doing something new.

Resistance means you're on the verge of a transformation—the more resistance, the bigger the transformational potential. So almost expect self-sabotage or resistance, and become aware of how it stops you from moving forward. Approach change with the thought of "*I wonder how my ego is going to try and stop me this time?*" And take note of all the creative ways your Ego or inner child interrupts your pattern of change.

Of course, there is a difference between self-sabotaging false resistance and real resistance when you're actually on the wrong path or making misaligned choices. Here's how you can tell the difference. If you are about to make a change that might be good for you, you may experience self-sabotage. In this instance, you are experiencing false resistance - or Egoic resistance. Your Ego is so afraid of changing that it tries to stop that change from happening. This self-sabotage generally occurs before or at the beginning of taking new action. This resistance can often dissipate while doing the new action, and you may feel great afterwards.

Here's an example of false resistance. You've started a new action, such as joining a dance class and resistance creeps in. You'll notice it because your mind will be filled with statements like, "I don't feel like going, maybe I'll start next week", or, "I'm too big to dance", or "I don't have the right shoes". Your mind will keep creating roadblocks. But, when you do finally go, you're only in resistance for the first 15 minutes before you realise how much fun you're having. You notice yourself leave lighter and happier. This early resistance is false resistance. It's just your Ego trying to stop you from creating changes or trying something new.

Real resistance is different. Let's say you've started your new action of going to a dance class. You're going consistently, but you don't enjoy it all, and you don't feel good afterwards. In this case, you may experience real resistance, letting you know that you are not on the right path and that this new action is misaligned for you. The feedback you will get from the Universe beyond these actions won't be very encouraging.

So how do you know you are on the right path?

One of the first things to note is that the Universe is constantly offering up signs and synchronicities to let us know that we are on the right path. The feedback we get back from the Universe provides a significant indication of whether we are on the right path or not.

At first, you may get some resistance; then, self-sabotage will try and stop you from creating any changes. Beyond resistance is the confusing Freeze phase. This is when we haven't achieved the full results yet, but we know it would be hard to go back to what we were. (Refer to my previous chapter, *Phases of change*. The Freeze phase is when you're already in the darkest part of the tunnel and are desperately trying to see the light at the end.)

Obviously, we prefer to stay in our comfort zone, but when we dare to move beyond that self-sabotaging Freeze phase and start taking new actions, we start getting some new results. At this point, you need to pay very close attention to feedback from the Universe.

Say, for example, you want to find a new job that's more aligned to you. You start taking action to reach this goal by sending out CVs, filling out applications and going for interviews. You may hear of a position that's become available. Someone might offer you another job you never considered, or you may land numerous job interviews. Still, none of these result in you actually getting the job. These are great signs!! These results tell you that you are on the right path, but you aren't there yet. You are slowly stepping into the vibration of someone aligned to a new job.

Here are some other examples: you want to go on a holiday and start attracting lots of holiday brochures or unexpected conversations with travel agents. Or you'd like to sell your house, and suddenly you start bumping into property consultants. These are all indications that your new actions are attracting results that are in alignment with your desire. It may still take more consistent new actions to get you to the end of the tunnel, the final outcome of your intention coming to fruition. Initially, some natural resistance can almost be seen as a bit of a test, just to see how badly you want your intention and how consistent you can be. This is not the place to give up.

Unfortunately, lots of people do give up! They become impatient or discouraged. If they want that new job but keep getting rejected, they withdraw and stop applying. They hide away to lick their wounds. If they don't sell their house, they take it off the market. These are ways of quitting and going back to their comfort zone. They essentially go back to square one and undo all the momentum they've created through their new actions. Then they have to start again. Ego has won; it pulled you back into old patterns.

This back and forth becomes incredibly exhausting on the body and its energetic state. Constantly stopping and starting puts your body in a constant state of anxiety, in anticipation of change. No real transformational results can take place when you are continually going back to the beginning. You deprive yourself of the ability to then stabilise in a new life. You never actually reach your goal.

The most important thing is to pay an incredible amount of attention to the feedback that the Universe is giving you. Generally, you will get new results or consequences to your actions within a few days of a new action you are taking. Don't change or course-correct too quickly or you risk cancelling out or not reaping the benefits of your new action. Stay the course, stay persistent, and if you see nothing new coming up for you within a few days, then try another new action. If you find that the action causes you real resistance, then you need to consider something else or taking different action steps.

False resistance doesn't last long; it just requires a little persistence. Generally, you will see some positive synchronicities within a few days. Real resistance continuously feels wrong over a long period and can attract negative synchronicities.

CHAPTER 19

Individuality vs collective consciousness

After watching the Matrix, I often joked, why not take the purple pill? No, I'm not encouraging anyone to take drugs! In the Matrix, there were only two options. Take the blue pill and go about your daily life as usual as a part of one big organism, functioning as an efficient hive mind (similar to what Eric Pepin from the Higher Balance Institute calls Red Cells). The other choice is the red pill. Take that and become aware and find out the truth about everything. Why only pick one? Combine them both, and you make the purple pill.

The one thing all of us humans have in common is that we all chose to have this human experience. We chose to experience the Matrix the way we are experiencing it now.

On a collective level, we are operating within a Hive mind or collective consciousness of sorts. All you have to do is look at the programming around you! There are patterns everywhere, and we rely on everyone to follow the rules to function as a society. If people didn't stop at red lights, it could create some bad outcomes. We need rules, structure and organisation. A hive mind helps ants build well-functioning colonies, bees build beehives and organised humans build cities.

On an individual level, our separation from the Hive defines who we are as individuals. We can be creative, self-expressive and do something unique that defines us from all others. On an individual level, we have a taste of freedom from the Hive and understand our unique personal power.

When you look at your TV, do you realise that there are thousands of pixels of light all organised together to create an image? If a pixel suddenly became conscious of itself and chose to break the pattern and fly off in a different direction, the TV programmer would think, "*Oh no, one of the cells has gone rogue!*" You may even throw the TV away. A programmer may view an individual cell that isn't conforming as a virus, prompting them to do everything possible to put the pixel back in place. It's the same when you are perceived to be doing something that could threaten the evolution of the collective. The universe might treat you like a virus and create ways to constantly pull you back into the Matrix programming of the collective mind.

You are that individual pixel on that screen, functioning as a part of a whole picture, as well as an individual being. If you choose to break out as an individual, you will set off the alarm bells and alert the programmer of this reality. Doing so would force the programmer to find ways to bring you back to your regular programming. That's how self-sabotage begins; when you've triggered the attention of the programmer. I'm speaking in metaphors but hoping you understand the concept.

The secret to the purple pill is that you have the knowledge of both! Know that you are a separate individual with the power to break free if you wanted to and know you are also part of a larger functioning system. Have the knowledge of both the blue pill and the red pill at the same time. It will give you an advantage over everyone else. You are one, and you are all. At the very least, you are awake!

If you pick only one pill, in essence, only one perspective, you become dormant to the perspective of the other.

Living from this place of knowledge, you are powerful because you've learnt how to function in a way that doesn't put you on the programmer's radar. You're not rebelling, you're following the rules. You can still influence your environment in subtle ways. The programmer won't sabotage what you do as long as you're not trying to create too many drastic changes to the system at once. You see, even the programmer fears change. Even the programmer has an Ego. Why else is the programmer doing its shadow work here in

3D form through us? We are the individual cells of the programmer itself.

The purple pill gives you the knowledge of everything to ultimately enjoy the simplicity of daily living in all its pain and joy, in full acceptance of everything you are. This is knowledge the programmer doesn't want you to have. By knowing that you have the free will to choose, the programmer suffers the risk of you rebelling and forcing the programmer into its own dark night of the soul, which would not be very fun for us littler cells. Can you imagine what a dark night of the soul would be like for Source? If we little human cells all decided to force Source into one huge phase of change? Imagine the turmoil for us little humans. Maybe it would end up like another Noah's Arc!

CHAPTER 20

To sum it all up

Humans struggle to awaken and stay awake due to their relationship with their emotions. The problem is that hormones and the endocrine system still drive us. We are programmed this way to ensure the survival of our species.

Dopamine makes you feel successful. Oxytocin makes you feel love. Serotonin stabilises your mood, and endorphins are natural pain killers. Hormones create comfortable emotions to aid in your physical 3D body's care and survival.

Your emotions are constantly hijacking your physical body. So the logical, rational thinking mind struggles to get through to us. We continue to react emotionally within every situation and lack clarity in our thinking. The most primitive part of the brain is in a constant preoccupation with our physical needs and our species' survival.

Some spiritual teachers say that women only have access to their truest clairvoyance skills and intuition when the hormonal need to have children or a deep connecting relationship no longer controls them. Often this is after menopause. Even if a child is born with these gifts of seeing, these gifts can either diminish or become completely impossible to control in the teenage years. This is due to the fluctuating hormone activity within the body.

More often, women who are settled, not seeking out a relationship or know that they no longer want to have any children or more children, are the women who seem to be the freest to access their higher intuition. When you are free from hormonal control and no longer triggered by the desire to search for external satisfaction, you can then look inwards for this satisfaction instead. When neediness no longer drives a woman, she is free to seek internal joy and satisfaction.

These confident, stabilised, independent women can reach enlightenment and access their spiritual gifts more readily, without the physical calling's distractions.

Are you still being controlled by your emotions? Is the biological system that you are currently animating hijacking your rational thinking mind? When a problem comes up that triggers an emotion within you, are you able to process and rationalise your thoughts, or do you get sucked into a snowball of emotions and reactions?

Now I'm not saying that emotions are wrong. Emotions play a crucial role in our physical survival. Emotions are necessary for our evolution because they are your internal guidance system telling you what feels right and what wrong. However, the world of spirit and energy doesn't understand emotions because they don't have hormones or an endocrine system. They only understand signature patterns or the vibrations that emotion causes. Emotions are simply a feature of the physical, biological, human body that we shed when we die. The realm of energy uses that energy we create from our emotions to charge up their ability to manifest and create at a physical 3D level.

Let's revisit a previous example that explains this manifestation/creation process. The world of energy/spirit/data downloads the inspiration to make a cake. Your physical, biological brain interprets this information, just like tapping into a radio signal, then translates it into the action of actually baking the cake. Presto! The world of energy just baked a cake through you!

I realise I'm spending a lot of time repeating this concept because I need you to understand it for the next and most important part of your learning.

We live in a Universe where the Law of Attraction is one of the laws we have to live by. It says that the energy that you create within you is the same energy you will attract back.

There are two basic types of energy, creative/construction energy and destructive energy. The lower groupings of emotions are destructive energy. The higher groups of emotions are constructive energy.

Suppose a person is operating from the lower emotional groupings. They take no personal responsibility and are a drain on society. They are giving this destructive energy to the spirit/energy world to work with. When a person acts in such a way, the world of energy can only guide you in destructive ways. It's like giving someone a shopping trolley with a wonky wheel. You have to work with what you get, and it may be a struggle. Spirit has to work with what you give them.

Now, if you operate from a place of courage, self-empowerment, love and compassion, you generate creative energy for the spirit realm to work with. Only good and creative construction can come from good creative energy. This is why it's so important that we learn how to harness our ability to use constructive energy rather than destructive energy. We must give the spirit realm the resources that we want to see and feel more of.

You can choose an emotion at will! Better yet, you can act on an emotion at will. In the lower groupings of emotions, such as the disempowering emotions and the controlling emotions, you are controlled by emotions. You are controlled by your human physical body and your endocrine system. Within the upper groups of emotions, the power emotions upwards, your higher self, your spirit self, has more say over your life. You can make a choice. Do you want your emotions to control you, or do you want to control your emotions? Control your emotions, and you have more control over your own physical experience. Knowing this secret is the key to a happy and successful life.

By activating the higher emotions, you are better able to rationalise a broader perspective. By activating and operating from the higher emotions, you can use discernment to determine which part of yourself gives more beneficial guidance.

Here's an example. If you lie down in the street and look up at a building, you get one perspective. Walk into the building and take the elevator half-way, and your perspective changes. If you go to the top of the building and stand on the ledge, this is a whole new perspective. Now you have the experience and knowledge of three perspectives. So how does this relate to emotions? You once knew what it was like to physically survive within all the lower emotions of fear, insecurity, shame, and sadness. As you worked your way up, you knew what it felt like to feel slightly better. You were able to have compassion for those in a lower state because you had been there.

If you are in constant sadness and depression, you can't know or understand the higher emotions of joy, peace, playfulness and perfection. It's too much of a leap in thinking from your limited lower perspective. It's like lying in the street and looking up at the building, trying to comprehend the view from the top when you've never seen it or experienced anything like it.

Let's make emotions work for us, not allow the emotions to control us. What emotion do you want to feel more of? Pick one! Any emotion that is the next level up from the primary emotions you've been operating from. Start to live, breathe, act from and make choices from that emotion. Do this for three to four weeks consistently.

Start to take notice of what type of feedback the Universe gives you. Use the emotion you choose as a building block and watch how the law of attraction works within the Universe. Notice how the Universe tries to repay you with that same emotion coming back to you. The Universe is an incredible feedback system.

Remember that no one can do this for you, and no one is stopping you. Only you can help yourself by choosing the emotions you wish to live by. You can create the life you desire with the awesome tool that is your emotions.

In the words of Anthony Robbins, "Emotion is a habit. We can train it like a muscle. Emotional fitness expands your thoughts, our understandings, our actions, our abilities, the way we interact with people and the way we experience the world."

So, where will you choose to live and operate from emotionally?

CHAPTER 21

Understanding Karma

Sadly, most people don't understand how Karma works and use it to explain why bad things happen to themselves or others. In reality, Karma is so much more complex than this, and it can be more liberating than you think.

No matter what you are doing, every minute of the day, you are making choices. It may be to sit on the couch, eat a particular food, ignore someone, overwork - everything you do. There is an energy behind every choice you make.

For example, imagine a friend asks you to meet up for a coffee. You really don't feel like going, but you say yes because you feel obligated. That sense of obligation will attract more situations into your life where you feel more of a sense of obligation.

This world is a physical mirror projection of what you choose. Karma simply turns your choices into a consequence so you can physically see what you are manifesting or creating.

The great news about this is that Karma serves us beautifully when we make positive choices. When you choose to act upon a positive emotion, Karma becomes highly protective of us. Making positive choices envelopes us in a very safe Karmic bubble. The universe will reflect back endless possibilities without us getting a scratch.

I know your next question, why does someone manifest abuse or an illness? In this case, a deeper investigation of the Karma playing out is needed. It may be related to family genetic choices, past life patterns or the collective consciousness/thinking into which a child is born. The less ability someone has to make choices for themselves, the more susceptible they are to the choices that the people around them are making.

When someone isn't able to make many choices for themselves and isn't taking any responsibility for their choices, they end up living out negative unjust Karma that isn't necessarily theirs. The sooner a person has the opportunity to take responsibility, accountability and control over their own choices, the sooner they can create their own Karma.

Have you ever wondered how some people can do the craziest things and get away with it? These people have generated and accumulated a lot of positive Karma. Remember that if you can't see a pattern, it doesn't mean that there isn't a pattern present.

When something negative happens, you often hear people say, "I must have attracted this", or, "They must have attracted what they got." You rarely see someone pat themselves on the back when something positive happens and say, "Yay me! I created that!"

It's great that a person takes responsibility for their choices because this is where the key to their power lies. But the critical distinction is to shift out of the pattern of victimisation, and move into a pattern of creating positive Karma, to empower you. It's your right to create the life you want through choice.

Once we become conscious of the ability to create through our own choices, life becomes a joyful experience, where you are no longer afraid of what can happen to you.

Accumulate and stay in positive Karma flow by making positive choices derived from positive, self-empowering emotions. The universe will go out of its way to protect you and give you everything you desire. That's the Law of Attraction.

CHAPTER 22

Save our emotions

The more you look at the direction society is going, the more you realise we are headed towards a world where emotions are not ok. You already know your parents and society suppressed most of your emotions from a young age. Those intellectual minds in power seem to say which emotions are too much, which amount of emotion is just enough and which ones are not ok.

Hollywood movies like Equals, Divergent, Hunger Games, Maze Runner, Equilibrium, The Giver and anything within the Zombie apocalypse genre are trying to warn humanity (I highly recommend all of these movies, by the way. Especially Equals). The warning is, *control your emotions or else.* Simply look at the school systems and how everyone is categorised. Conform and fit in, or else you will be separated from those you love. You risk never being allowed to feel again. You risk being medicated or locked away. You risk living in a society where giving up your life is ok, and no one will care if you do. If you become over-emotional, then you can't fit in.

If humans continue to be careless with their emotions or if they continue to use them as an excuse to hurt, rape, kill, steal and remove others' free will, we will be stripped of them. They will be taken away because they are unsafe for society.

In the meantime, while they try to find ways to suppress your emotions, the next best thing is to separate you from society. People who can't control their emotions will be put with people who are out of control of their emotions. Only those who can manage their emotions will be able to live freely within society.

In my opinion, society needs to be focussing more on teaching people how to feel and express their emotions safely, rather than suppressing them. Emotions need to be accepted as a part of us. Emotions need to be ok, and suppressing them is not an option. They are tools used by your physical self and your higher mind self to communicate with one another.

Imagine for a moment being stripped of your emotions. Imagine not being able to feel the skin on your child's face or dancing and feeling the music. Imagine not being able to enjoy the taste of your favourite food or having the pleasure of making love. If you have to be separated from society because you can't control your emotions, what's the point of being in a physical body? If you aren't allowed to feel emotions, and you're not allowed to learn what feelings are, what's the point of your higher self animating your physical body? You can only have feelings if you have a physical body. The world of spirit or energy is clueless to what touch is or what a kiss feels like because it's a construct of the physical 3D experience. Our higher self is learning what feelings and emotions are through this physical existence.

If we don't learn how to stop hurting ourselves and each other, we are most definitely headed towards a future society where emotions won't be allowed. So, what can we do about it? We need to learn how to use our emotions as a tool for good and connection, not negativity and separation. We need to learn to guide and assist our emotions. We need to prove that our emotions don't control us in order for their control to be left up to us.

Our 3D, 4D and 5D self are constantly interacting and co-creating with each other. We are continually creating on all dimensions. If you want to change an emotion, you need to change it at a 3D physical level through actions or our basic five senses, at a 4D level through your feelings and emotions and at a 5D level through your rational and logical thinking. We must get all dimensions working together by making sure they are all producing behaviour, actions, emotions, feelings and thoughts that align with each other. For example, if you love your partner, behave as though you love them. Choose actions that show you love them. Touch them as though you love them. Express feelings that show this love. Create thoughts centred on your love for them. You must get all dimensions of yourself on board with your love for them. There is no room for doubting your love for them.

If you want to be more self-loving, you can't claim that you love and value yourself yet behave and act in ways that contradict this. These actions include feeling unloved, having unloving thoughts about yourself or making unloving choices for yourself. It would be best if you lived your intentions and emotions truly. Whichever emotion you choose to focus on, you need to focus it into all dimensions of your existence. Work diligently and be self-disciplined on this. Practice the ability to play with your emotions and feel them in every way you can without hurting others. We are collectively fighting for our rights to keep our emotions. Help humanity, help save our emotions.

Higher levels of consciousness from 7D upwards are different. At this level, it's more about being rather than doing. However, it seems that humanity hasn't yet mastered what it is doing yet.

So, let's leave the beingness of 7D upwards for another book, shall we? I give you a little clue, 7D is all about relationships, interactions and how we connect with others. In 7D, there is little to no separation or free will. We are one. Therefore, to live in a 7D state of consciousness is to accept everything and everyone as one with you, even your enemies and those you fear.

My advice? Master your 3D to 6D first. Leave the 7D for when you've taken care of your own backyard first.

Love and light to you on your journey!
Carla Savannah

Other Books by Carla Savannah

How Do I Know When I'm Ready to Have Kids?
The Spiritual Awakening of a Spray Tanner
21st Century Relationships

Available for purchase at
www.carlasavannah.com.au

www.ingramcontent.com/pod-product-compliance
Lightning Source LLC
Chambersburg PA
CBHW072135020426
42334CB00018B/1812